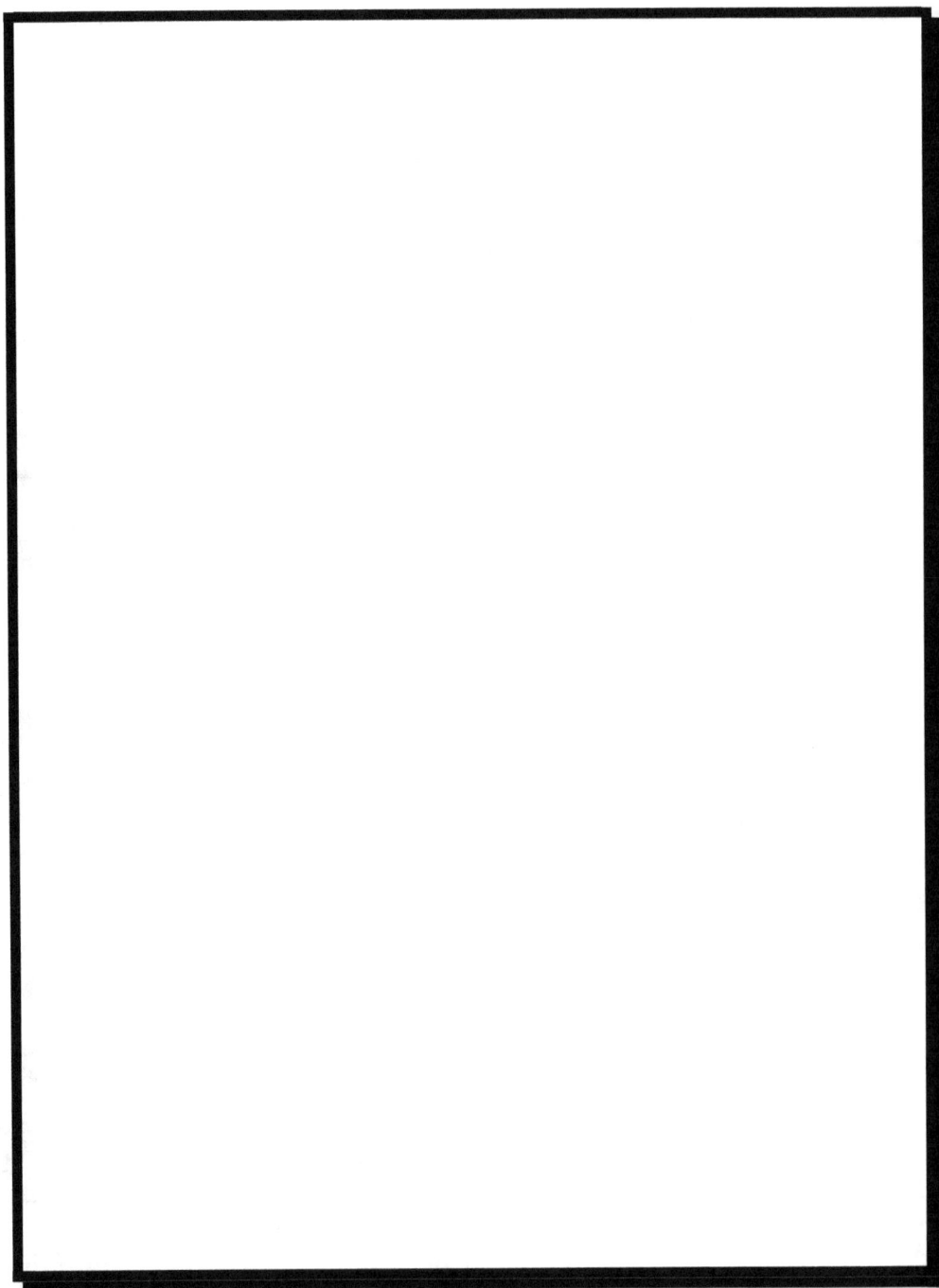

SAVING YOUR HAIR STRANDS ONE AT A TIME!

SAVING YOUR HAIR STRANDS ONE AT A TIME

"What Some Stylist Won't Tell You, but I Will"

Your Guide To Achieving A Healthy Head of Hair!!!

By

Erica Turner

Saving Your Hair Strands One At A Time! What Some Stylist Won't Tell you, but I Will!

By Erica Turner

Printed in the United States of America

Copyright © 2015 Erica Turner

ISBN#: 13:978-0692577851

ISBN: 13:978-069257781
Healthier Hair, Treatments, Color, Heat Damage,
Shampoo, Conditioners, Alopecia

HELPFUL HINTS

In this instructional guide, I will provide for you what I believe are helpful tips and techniques to accomplish a beautiful healthy head of hair.

SAVING YOUR HAIR STRANDS ONE AT A TIME *is an awesome guide for all. This guide will teach you how to search for a life time stylist as well as the dos and don'ts of home maintenance for your hair. You will find tips for products, treatments, personal hair care and more. After reading this guide you will have the knowledge of how to **SAVE YOUR HAIR STRANDS ONE AT A TIME.***

DEDICATION

In memory of my grandfather (John Paul)

In memory of my grandmother (Maggie)

In honor of my father (Eddie)

In honor of my mother (Mary)

In honor of my stepfather (Willis)

In honor of my children

Markeita

Shantesia

Caleb

Destiny

In honor of my sister (Kim)

In honor of my niece (Zaria)

In honor of my aunts (Ann) (Lisa)

In honor of my uncle (John Edward)

In honor of my uncle (Sammy)

In honor of my cousins (Shondra) (Quita)

I LOVE YOU ALL!

SAVING YOUR HAIR STRANDS ONE AT A TIME

ACKNOWLEDGEMENTS

First I would like to Thank God for giving me the strength to pursue all of my dreams and passions. In spite of numerous setbacks; as my foundation, God has allowed me to endure through them all, and for that I am eternally grateful!

SPECIAL THANKS: *To Barbara Edmonds, The best teacher a stylist such as I could ever have. You've instilled in me knowledge that I'll cherish for a lifetime. Thank you for simply being there.*

SPECIAL THANKS: *To my encourager, my prayer warrior, my example of strength, and one who loves the Lord my mother, I Love You!*

CONTENTS

INTRODUCTION

Hair, for some women, is like the covering of her life. This is felt by the majority of women in the world. A good hair day can make the worst day a little brighter. There is a sense of confidence and self-esteem we get as women when our hair is healthy and beautiful.

I pray that this book will teach and guide you in accomplishing all of your goals when it comes to the health of your hair. It is my mission to help as many women as possible achieve and embrace the natural beauty of their hair. Regardless of hair style choice, whether it's natural or relaxed there is a remedy to achieve a healthy state.

CHAPTER ONE

What Is Hair?

....

A perfect beginning is to understand what hair is. The definition of hair is any threadlike strands growing from the skin of humans, mammals, and other animals. It's a protein thread-like fiber also known as (Keratin). The outer structure of hair is composed of Keratin. These are fibrous proteins that are the main structural component of hair and nails. Hair is all over the body, but the scalp being the most noticeable area. Hair grows about half an inch a month for most people. However, this is dependent upon genetics, age, and hormonal changes. Any of these changes may affect the rate of hair growth at any given time. The healthier the cuticle layer is the better chance you have of growing healthier and longer hair. Each strand of hair is made up of 3 layers. The first layer is the cuticle layer which is the most important because it is the protective layer. The better you take care of this layer the stronger the hair will become. The second layer is the cortex. The cortex is where everything enters through the cuticle from water, shampoo, conditioners and chemicals. When the cuticle layer is damaged, the hair will become weak, dry, brittle, stiff, and hard to manage. This is when conditioner treatments come into play because when the cuticle layer is conditioned properly it protects the cortex. We will discuss conditioners in another chapter. The last layer is the medulla. Its function is not absolutely clear, and sometimes this layer is absent in some types of hair. The cuticle, being the first and most important layer, is the layer that protects the cortex which is the inner layer (second layer). When using colors or chemicals, this layer is where change takes place. The way you protect this layer is by keeping a well-conditioned cuticle layer. Medulla the third layer, remember some have them some don't. When this layer is present the hair tends to be softer and has more ability to hold moisture. Picture 1A shows us a hair strand from the inside out. The cortex is located outside of the medulla and the cuticle is on the outside of the cortex which means it surrounds both the cortex and the medulla. Picture 1B shows us the surface of the cuticle layer. On the left it indicates what a healthy strand looks like under the microscope and on the right it shows you what a damaged cuticle looks like. Remember this is what it looks like when the cortex is exposed.

Surface of Hair - Cuticle

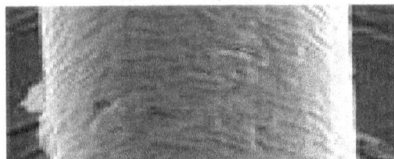

* Virgin/Healthy Hair

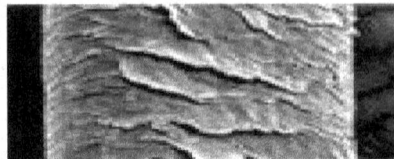

* Damaged Hair

1B

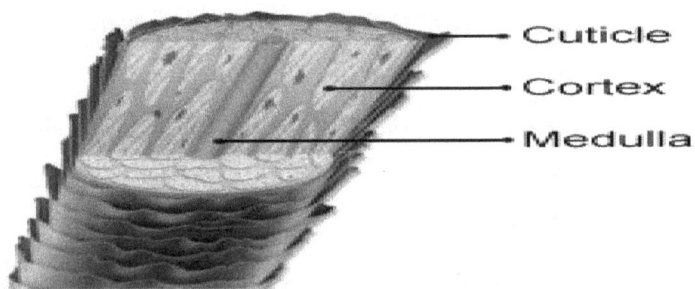

Cuticle

Cortex

Medulla

1A

CHAPTER TWO

Which Shampoo & Conditioner Are Best For Me?

....

In this industry we have a very big variety of shampoos and conditioners. When you ask, which shampoo is for you, you first have to ask yourself what your hair needs or what is it lacking. There are important factors to consider:

Is your hair oily, dry, brittle, and fine? Do you have product build-up or do you just need a good cleansing shampoo? Once you understand your hair and what it needs, you're able to choose a shampoo properly. There are different types of shampoos, but first let's start with a clarifying shampoo. This shampoo should be used when a deep cleanse is desired. It helps remove build-up, chlorine, oil, medication and other things that could be harmful to the hair and scalp. Always make sure you read the labels on all your shampoos and conditioners to make sure it's what you actually need before you purchase it. After using a clarifying shampoo, I always suggest you follow behind with a moisturizing shampoo, because clarifying shampoos tend to strip the hair of its natural oils. This shampoo is designed to supplement and replenish the hair's natural oils, which is really needed if your hair lacks moisture and is very dry. In order to restore moisture you would need to choose a shampoo that cleanses and moisturizes the hair and scalp without removing your hair's natural oils. The lack of moisture could be caused by environmental changes, products, heat, and personal care. On the other hand oily hair is different, but when dealing with African Americans nine times out of ten we're not dealing with oily hair. Another thing you would want to do is avoid using oils and grease. You may also want to shampoo more on a weekly basis. For instance, if you usually shampoo once every two weeks try once or twice a week to see if that helps. The other three types of shampoos I would like to mention are Dandruff Shampoo, Neutralizing Shampoo, and Color-Treated Shampoos. These three are exactly what they say they are. Dandruff Shampoo is for dandruff which means this is a medicated formula shampoo. Its job is to remove dry or oily flakes from the scalp. It is not designed to be used on a daily basis, but can be used on a regular basis to help treat and remove dandruff. If you have any serious issues like eczema or severe dandruff I recommend you seek a professional dermatologist for treatment. Sometimes they will prescribe a shampoo for you which you should always take to your stylist at every salon visit. Color-treated shampoos are designed for color treated hair. You have some shampoos when it comes to color that are specifically designed for gray, blonde, or even red colors. These shampoos are to be said formulated with extra conditioning agents to help with the longevity of the color. Hate to say this but, from my experience sometimes they work and sometimes they don't. If you choose a good moisturizing conditioning shampoo which was mentioned earlier then you should be fine. Best choice is to use professional products that cater to your hair needs. The last shampoo I would like to mention is the neutralizing shampoo. This shampoo is designed to be used with your relaxer services. I have heard people say they use a regular shampoo or whatever they may have at home lying around. Please don't do this. The main purpose for neutralizing shampoo is to stop the action of the chemical (relaxer). This specific shampoo actually neutralizes caustic or alkali residue that's in the hair. If this is not done, then the chemical will continue to work even after you've styled your hair causing chemical burns and sometimes hair loss. Neutralizing shampoo should only be used when a relaxer service has been given. Please for all relaxer services seek a professional stylist. Now let's talk conditioners. Conditioners are used to help restore the hair and keep it in a healthy state. We have conditioners that are penetrating conditioners which mean it reaches deep down into that cortex layer which is your second layer that was mentioned in chapter one. These are used to restore protein and, most of the time these types of conditioners are used for treatments to help strengthen and rebuild damaged and weaken hair by placing the client under the dryer with a plastic cap for 10-15 minutes. Now for your ever day conditioners this is referred to as a non-penetrating conditioner. Which means it only coats the cuticle layer. The best quality of conditioners will coat leaving a microfilm coating. This helps prevent static, protects the cuticle layer, and helps the hair to be healthier and stronger. Other conditioners are reconstructors, protein packs or special treatments. These should be used only when needed and directions should be followed very carefully because some of them are very concentrated and at the end of the day even though we need protein sometimes when misused or used too much it could result in damage. The last conditioner I would like to mention is a Leave-In Conditioner. This is just what it says leave-in. Some of these conditioners have great benefits. They have taken things a little further by providing extra moisture, and proteins to help strengthen the hair even after it's styled. Yes believe it or not it continues to work days after it's been applied. Also leave-ins work very well as detanglers, and provide a good layer of protection from heat styling. It's a good idea to add this to your home maintenance especially if you use a lot of heat on your hair. When using conditioners, always remember that, there is such a thing as over conditioning. This happens when one is conditioning too much. I know you're saying wow, you can actually condition too much. Yes and when this happens your hair becomes limp, heavy, and weighed down. In other words it will not move. I mean no blowing in the wind what so ever (Laughs). Please ladies keep these things in mind when caring for your strands.

CHAPTER THREE

What Causes Heat Damage

....

There are several things that cause heat damage. We all know the famous Flat Iron that is so popular these days. They come in various sizes, colors, and temperature settings, but don't let that fool you! The flat iron, along with blow dryers and curling irons can all cause heat damage when used on a regular basis. When purchasing these tools you must check for quality. This doesn't mean you have to spend lots of money, but it would be a good idea to research the tool that you're thinking about purchasing before you actually purchase it. It's not a good idea to use these tools on a day to day basis. When it comes to natural hair, signs of heat damage will began to show after a good shampoo. It will show in the curl pattern while wet. The curl pattern will either return to its natural curl pattern, or if damaged, it will be slightly or extremely altered. It could appear to be curly in one area, tighter in another and just straight on the ends. This is due to extremes amount of heat from these tools. Excessive heat could also cause split ends as well as breakage. This will cause your strands to feel dry, ruff, and appear to be dull. Once this happens, it is imperative to remove those ends. If those split ends are not removed, it could travel all the way to the top of that hair strand. This in the end will be much more damaging. It's always good to have your ends trimmed at least once every two months or at every relaxer service if needed. These tools could be very damaging! Please research information about tools such as these before purchasing them for home use. Your hair stylist will be a great person to get advice in regards to styling tools. This could save you a lot of time and money! Here are a few pointers when looking for a great styling appliance:

Does it have a display and control knob for temperature settings? A good tool will have this listed. It's always best to purchase tools that you can control the temperature. Some settings vary form 175 – 450 settings and yes we know that everybody wants silky straight hair but using any tool for home maintenance at 400 on a day to day basis is just dangerous! Yet you have people doing it and get upset when their hair begins to reflect the damage that has been done. Ladies it's evident that these tools could cause serious damage. Please minimize the usage of these tools to minimize damage.

CHAPTER FOUR

How Can I Prevent Shedding & Breakage

....

As we know we shed at least 40 to 80 strands per day. Some people get scared when they see a few strands here and there. Well I'm here to tell you that, that's ok. No need to worry! Always keep in mind that it's most common to shed more in the fall and winter than any other time unless you're experiencing other problems. This is due to seasonal and environmental changes. During these months we tend to have drier skin as well as scalp because of the cold air and harsh winds. When the leaves began to change you may notice change in your skin. It becomes dry rough and even itches sometimes. Well your scalp reacts the same way, and when this happens it causes the hair to become dry as well. Because of this dryness the hair strands become weak. It's just like a plant. If you notice when you water a plant and give it the right amount of sunlight it produces beautiful leaves; as soon as you stop giving it water and letting it get that light the leaves become dry and weak. If not watered in enough time, they will become completely dry and fall off. Once watered and exposed to sunlight the leaves begin to sprout again. Well your hair and scalp are the same way, but it's very important to moisturize and hydrate your hair and scalp before this happens! You may do this by doing deep conditioner treatments as well as hot oil treatments. The oil is to keep the scalp lubricated and protect it from the dryness. The deep conditioner will penetrate deep into the cortex layer to provide strength and help protect the hair from shedding and breakage. These are two things that you can always do regardless of the season, but it will be more needed during these times. Another way to prevent shedding keep your ends trimmed as mentioned in the previous chapter. Some people really don't think that trims are very important. I can't emphasize it enough but it's so important to the point where it makes a difference between a trim and a cut. It's like if you had a tree with a damaged branch that you refuse to cut off it begins to affect the whole tree. Please cut those bad branches off! It's better to lose a branch than to lose the whole tree. Ladies Let's Save These Hair Strands One At A Time!

CHAPTER FIVE

Medication, Hair Loss & Alopecia

....

Hair loss and Alopecia are very scary topics, but they affect many people each and every day. When we as women began to lose our hair it becomes very stressful, depressing and overwhelming at times. We may find ourselves wondering what did we do or what did we use that maybe causing the hair loss? One factor could be medications that you are taking. Some medications cause hair loss. Sometimes doctors don't even mention hair loss as a side effect to a medication that they've just prescribed to you. It is your full responsibility as a patient to ask courageous questions and to research side effects on medication that has been prescribed to you. Besides medication, they're also other reasons we could experience hair loss. For instance, stress itself could cause temporary hair loss, and that could be double trouble if your medication is already affecting your hair. It's so many illnesses and diseases that affect our hair and we never even realize it. More issues that may cause hair loss are pregnancies, too much vitamin A, vitamin B deficiency, lack of protein, female hormones, hypothyroidism, anemia, Lupus, dramatic weight loss, chemotherapy, hereditary and other variables not listed here. Even though Alopecia is hair loss, it has different categories. One of the most common forms of alopecia is Traction Alopecia. This is a form of alopecia or gradual hair loss caused by persistent pulling, wearing tight ponytails or braids. Alopecia Areata is an autoimmune condition which causes patchy hair loss. It can result in a single bald patch or extensive patchy hair loss. In this case, the immune system attacks the hair follicles causing hair loss. However, this is not contagious. It mostly occurs in healthy individuals causing them to seek further care. Another common form of alopecia is Androgenetic Alopecia. This is known as male pattern baldness or female pattern baldness. It may cause thinning of the hair in both sexes. It is said to be hereditary and is the most progressive type of hair loss. There are plenty of other types of alopecia, but the ones I've named are some of the most common ones. Listed below are some of the other types just to share:

Scarring Alopecia, Ciatricial Alopecia, Alopecia Totalis and Alopecia Universalis. When we talk about Alopecia the list of different kinds could go on and on. So I say to you if you are experiencing any type of hair loss it's best to seek a professional doctor or dermatologist to get to the root of whats causing your issues. As we know, when you hear the word chemotherapy, we automatically think of hair loss due to the side effects of the treatments. Chemotherapy drugs are powerful medications that attack growing cancer cells, but unfortunately as a result, the medications also attack other growing cells in your body. This includes your hair roots. It may even cause hair loss all over the body not just the scalp. It includes your eyebrows, lashes, armpits, and more private Areas. Depending on the degree of the dosage of the medication, it could cause complete baldness or just thinning. Never feel embarrassed or be afraid to ask questions. Always remember that the only crazy or stupid question is the one that you never asked. If you or someone you may know has been diagnosed with cancer, please feel free to use/share the links below. These sites include information about support groups that could help as you or someone you know are experiencing the different changes in your life:

- American Cancer Society (www.cancer.org)
- Breast Cancer Group (www.breastcancer.org)
- Ovarian Cancer Group (www.ovariancancer.org)
- Cancer Support Groups (www.cancercare.org)

CHAPTER SIX

UNDERSTANDING GRAY & COLOR

....

As a professional stylist, I have been overwhelmed by the number of clients in my chair with different shades of green hair. Understanding gray is not that difficult if you have been taught the dos and the don'ts. The job of a professional stylist is to understand the chemistry behind the magic. As hair grows and forms, the pigment cells called melanocytes injects the hair with color. Melanocytes may also be referred to as (melanin), the color maybe blonde, brown, or red. As we age the production of melanin decreases, when it comes to a complete stop that's when we become completely gray. For some people it may never completely stop causing them to have salt and pepper color. So what we call gray hair is really just hair with no pigment. Gray hair can really be tricky when it comes to coloring. Some hairs are stiff and wiry being difficult to curl or color. This is where your professional comes in because as professionals we know how to treat the hair to get it to soften up so that it will take color better with a lasting result.

SAVING YOUR HAIR STRANDS ONE AT A TIME

The problem I see the most as a stylist is when an individual has tried to color their hair and it ends up green! Another observation I have witnessed is when the color fades, they have a different color other than gray. This is due to the hair grabbing the color of their choice base color. If you have not been taught color you will not understand color bases and what color to use to cancel out unwanted color or tones. Understanding how to mix, how much to mix, how long to process is essential for the best results. Color itself could cause some damage to the hair as well. When choosing color, one must know the differences between the different types of colors. You have henna colors, semi-permanent, demi-permanent, temporary and permanent colors. If you have not studied or been taught correctly about color, then you are headed for disaster! A $4.99 bottle of color from the beauty supply store could cause you a salon visit for $180 or more just for a corrective color. When it comes to the different types of colors mentioned before they all have different effects. Henna color is made from a plant. It is used for hair color and temporary body art work. This powdered color will activate with air and water once it's mixed. Then it becomes a paste and you may apply it directly to your hair or skin. When applied to the skin it becomes a temporarily tattoo, but when it's applied to the hair it becomes a permanent hair color. The difference between semi-permanent and temporary hair colors are that one lasts longer than the other. Temporary color rinses out after one shampoo. It comes in a spray, hair mascara, or a color-depositing shampoo. Semi-permanent hair colors last from 6-12 shampoos. These are used when you would like to darken your hair or tone because it has no lifting power. When wanting the color to have a longer lasting effect such as women with gray, then demi-permanent color will be a better choice. Demi-permanent, like Semi-permanent colors, darkens and intensifies your natural or highlighted hair color, but longevity is 12-24 shampoos. When desiring a more permanent change then that's when permanent color is your best option. Permanent hair color changes your hair color, but remains until it has grown completely out or it has been removed by cutting. My advice for color is the same for chemicals: always seek a professional first.

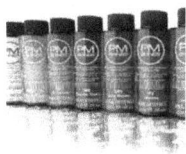

Demi-Permanent

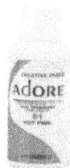

Semi-Permanent

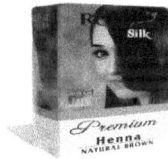

Henna

Temporary Hair Color

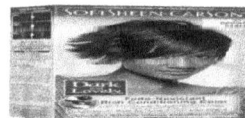

Permanent Hair Color

CHAPTER SEVEN

Sodium Hydroxide Verses Calcium Hydroxide

....

There are different types of Hydroxide relaxers. Hydroxide relaxers include Sodium Hydroxide, Potassium Hydroxide, Guanidine Hydroxide and Lithium Hydroxide. These relaxers are marketed and sold as Lye and No Lye or Base and no Base relaxers. In Lye relaxers the main ingredient is Sodium Hydroxide. This type of relaxer breaks down the hair bonds quickly which causes the hair to become straight. Licensed professionals are trained to perform this chemical service in a timely manner according to the client's hair texture, sensitivity of their scalp and the directions of the manufacture of the product being used. One must be careful when using this product because one common side effect of this product is scalp burning. If not applied properly and in a timely manner, one may suffer scalp burning even if the correct relaxer for your hair texture was chosen. This could actually lead to hair loss. Now even though all relaxers could cause some hair loss, Sodium Hydroxide relaxers are the most commonly used by professionals today. With that being stated, please allow a professional to apply this product. Without the proper training, application and knowledge, one may start with a full head of hair and end up with none. Keep in mind that these relaxers have the same chemical as Drano (a product used to unclog pipes through dissolving material that is causing blockage) and some hair removal products. Relaxers are strong enough to remove your hair completely from your head! So before you decide to take this to your kitchen table and apply it to yourself, friends, or a family member, please seek a professional first! When it comes to different strengths these relaxers come in mild, regular, super, or normal strengths. This is what determines the amount or level of hydroxide used. Just for example a mild relaxer will have less Sodium Hydroxide than a regular or super relaxer. So when choosing which one is for you, there're many things one must take in consideration. There also No-Lye Relaxers. These relaxers fall under Lithium, Guanidine, Calcium and Potassium. Some are relaxers that you have to mix two ingredients together in order to make it active. The two ingredients are a cream containing Calcium Hydroxide and an activating solution which is called guanidine carbonate. In my own personal opinion and experience I dislike these types of relaxers because the most common side effects of this type of relaxer are drier

SAVING YOUR HAIR STRANDS ONE AT A TIME

hair which leads to sheading and breaking. This comes from the buildup of calcium on the hair. The best way this type of issue is corrected is for you to have regular salon visits to see your stylist for treatments to prevent this build up. I've had little girls sit in my chair and from just looking at their hair I can tell that their parents have been using these types of relaxers on their babies. When I ask the parents they say what YES! This is done because somewhere there were misunderstandings or a lack of knowledge of the damage these relaxers may cause. Believe it or not, the marketing of these products as no-lye or kiddie relaxers is a lie! I'm setting the record straight now! There is no such thing as kiddie relaxers, perm or whatever you want to call it. The pH balance for no-lye relaxers range from 9-11 and lye relaxers range from 12-14 whereas our hair is 4.5 - 5.5. If you place either or on hair, that pH is 4.5 - 5.5 to a 9 - 11 or 12 - 14 is putting the hair in danger, if you don't know what you're doing. Note to parents: Please get professional help when it comes to these chemicals. Always remember knowledge is what? POWER!

CHAPTER EIGHT

Why Isn't It Growing?

....

This is a question so often asked. Why isn't my hair growing? My answer is its growing. The only way your hair isn't growing is, you're either cutting it, it's falling out due to poor maintenance or it's something dealing with your health that may require medical attention. Other than that your hair should be growing. In order to grow, the hair has to be feed by something. The blood vessels are responsible for supplying nourishment to the hair and this happens at the base of the follicle. Hair grows from the follicle (root) which is located underneath the skin. Hair growth has three different phases. (ACT) Anagen, Catagen, and Teleogen. In each phase something different takes place. In the first phase, Anagen, the hair is growing. This is considered to be the (Growing Phase). The Anagen phase lasts about two to seven years. During this phase the length is determined. The second phase is called Catagen. In this phase the hair is transitioning so this is known as the (Transitioning Phase). This is the shortest phase only lasting about ten days. During this phase, the hair follicle actually shrinks and detaches itself from what we call the dermal papilla. After this has happened the hair begins its last phase which is the Teleogen phase. This is the phase of hair resting (Resting Phase). As new hair begins to grow, old hair is resting. In this phase

SAVING YOUR HAIR STRANDS ONE AT A TIME

at least 15% of the hair is going through the phase at the same time. This phase lasts about two to three months. Always remember that this is a repeating cycle it never ends it's an ongoing process. This is why it's always growing unless you are experiencing something that has interrupted this process. There are some diseases, deficiencies, and disorders that will cause an interruption in this cycle. If you think that you are or may be experiencing any of the deficiencies and disorders mentioned in chapter five that causes hair loss please seek medical attention as soon as possible. Some of these deficiencies and disorders if caught in time are treatable and reversible.

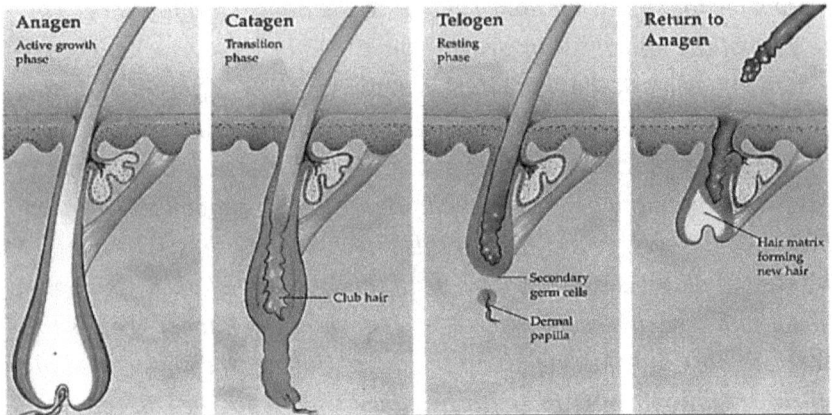

CHAPTER NINE

WHAT STYLIST IS FOR ME?

....

Ladies when choosing the best stylist for you, always look at these 5 key points.

- *Do they take continuing education classes, attend seminars or hair shows?*
- *Are they concerned about the health of your hair or your money?*
- *Do they tell you when something is wrong?*
- *How are their customer service skills?*
- *Do they educate you?*

A stylist that educates themselves constantly by attending seminars, hair shows and other continuing education classes, are pretty passionate about what they do. When it comes to something you love to do, a person will invest the extra time and money to build their skills. Whatever you're passionate about that's what you go hard for day in and day out. When you find a stylist that has this drive and passion for what they do, you've found you a stylist for a life time!

SAVING YOUR HAIR STRANDS ONE AT A TIME

This drive will also show in their work. They will always put their creative minds to work in order to give you the best of what they have. Nine times out of ten, you will leave their salon feeling renewed! Once they're behind the chair, it becomes a whole different ball game. Your hair then becomes their number one priority at that time. A true stylist understands that they must be focused on their job in order to know if there's anything going on with your hair, and being unfocused will probably cause them to miss something that might be very important. When searching for a stylist, you should look at their customer service skills. Do they seem well educated? Do they return calls, and texts, in a timely manner? When they book appointments do they over book or do they prioritize their time wisely? Do they hold a whole conversation on what they did the night before on their cell phones while performing your service? Do they lack when it comes to sharing with you about changes that they see taking place with your hair? If so, keep searching because that's not the stylist for you. You'll probably end up spending your whole day in the salon with them. These are just some of the important things you should look for when searching for a stylist. Make sure you can trust that your stylist will tell you the truth if they notice any thinning, shedding or breakage of your hair. Just like you have untruthful people around you every day don't exclude stylist from that list. Build trust with your stylist just like you build trust with your doctor. You trust your doctor with your life so you need to trust your stylist with your hair. Finding a stylist that cares can be a difficult task, but when you find one stick with them as long as your needs are being meet, your happy and your hair is healthy. Trust me chair hopping from stylist to stylist could cause you more damage in the end than in the beginning. If you have a stylist that doesn't have these key points you better run like your life depends on it (Laughing) cause even though your life doesn't your hair does!

CHAPTER TEN

NATURALS

....

Seems like in today's society natural hair is the thing to do. Well for some it's good and for others it's not. If you're considering going natural, it would be a good idea to speak with your stylist first. You and your stylist will be able to come up with the best plan for you while you're in transition. Going from relaxed hair to natural hair or vice versa could be very challenging. One may experience extreme breakage and shedding while others may not. It is very imperative that one condition's very well while natural. This is due to the lack of moisture that natural hair tends to have. I personally believe that natural hair is not for everyone. They're many things to take into consideration when considering going natural. The most important things are texture, the health of the strands and the person's ability to maintain a healthy natural state. While in transition their many different safe and healthy styles you could choose from. A lot of people choose to wear their strands in a sleek, silky look, which is called a Silk

Blow Out. This service is one of my favorites to perform, but I also inform my clients that too much heat is also not good. It's best to switch up sometimes, and do wet sets, twist outs, sew-ins, or even braids just to give your hair a break from the heat. I personally would not suggest putting heat on your hair every day. As mentioned before in chapter three, heat can cause just as much damage as a relaxer. Other things to consider before going natural are, do you sweat a lot and do you visit the gym frequently. If so it might just be even more challenging for you than others, but it is still achievable. Natural hair, once maintained and controlled is one of the most beautiful things one could ever wear.

References

1. *How quickly does hair grow?" 01 April 2000.*

HowStuffWorks.com<ins>http://health.howstuffworks.com/skin-care/hair-care/scalp-treatments/question251.htm</ins> 30 December 2015.

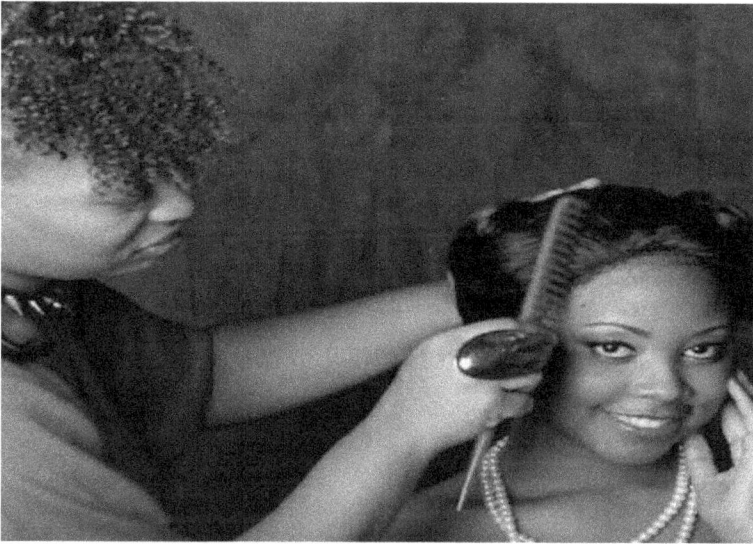

Author: Erica Turner

Model: Geri Alicea

ABOUT THE AUTHOR

Erica Turner is a single mother of four and a true entrepreneur. Holding the titles as a Licensed Cosmetologist, Colorist, Silk Out Artist, Product Owner, Educator, and now Author. She began her career as a braider at a young age in 2003, and then later obtained her Cosmetology License in February of 2009. After receiving her license in 2009, she wasted no time making a name for herself in the industry. Having the opportunity to work Bronner Brothers Hair Show in Atlanta, GA February of 2011, and 2015 she worked with some of the greatest in the industry including Lachelle Wise, Barber Edmonds, and James Mack just to name a few. As her passion continues to grow as a stylist and educator please look forward to more upcoming events from this highly driven entrepreneur.

(ENCOURAGING WORDS)

The saying goes the sky is the limit! Well I beg to differ. How can we say we serve God if we limit ourselves? Never limit yourselves and never allow anyone else too. I encourage you to aim and aim high! You never know how great you are unless you try. Whatever it is you want to accomplish in life, you can do it!

"We serve a Game Changing God so therefore there are NO LIMITS"

Quoted By

(Erica Turner)

GLOSSARY

Alopecia; The partial complete absence of hair from areas of the body where it normally grows; baldness.

Anagen; The first step in the hair growth cycle lasting about 3-7 years in human scalp hair.

Canities; The diminishing of pigment in hair producing a range of colors from normal to white that is perceived as gray. (Gray Hair)

Catagen; The brief portion of the hair cycle, in which the hair growth stops and begins to rest.

Cosmetologist; A beauty professional that is educated in treating hair, skin, and nails.

Calcium Hydroxide; A chemical compound with a variety of industrial and environmental uses.

Conditioner; A hair care product that changes the texture and appearance of the hair. Conditioners are viscous liquid, which is applied to the hair after shampooing.

Follicle; A mammalian skin organ that produces hair.

Hair; A protein filament that grows from follicles found in the dermis or skin.

Telogen; Known as the resting phase in the hair growth cycle. This phase lasts from 5-7 weeks.

Shampoo; A hair care product typically in the form of a viscous liquid that is used for cleaning hair.

Sodium Hydroxide; Sometimes referred to as lye. It is a chemical compound with a high alkaline content.

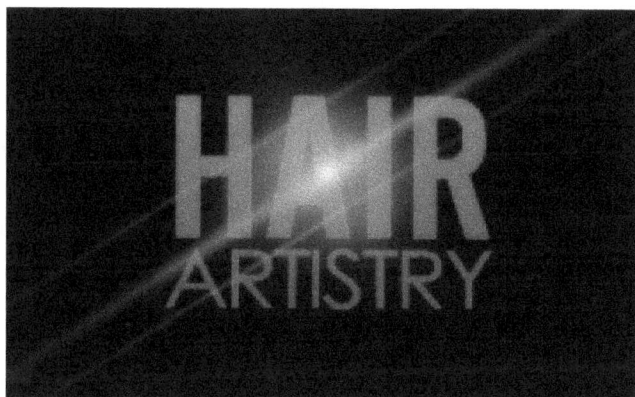

HAIR ARTISTRY PRODUCTS

Hair Artistry Deep Cleansing Shampoo 8oz $9.95

Hair Artistry Intensive Conditioner 8oz $10.95

Hair Artistry Leave-In Conditioner 8oz $11.95

To purchase visit www.HAProducts.bigcartel.com

SAVING YOUR HAIR STRANDS ONE AT A TIME

PG 39

SAVING YOUR HAIR STRANDS ONE AT A TIME

SAVING YOUR HAIR STRANDS ONE AT A TIME

SAVING YOUR HAIR STRANDS ONE AT A TIME